Living in the Lymelight

JENNY HODGES

DEDICATION

To every brave person battling a chronic health condition.
Take a moment and be proud of the strength that you show.
Never give up.

CONTENTS

AUTHOR'S NOTE

I've often been told I should write my story and not being a keen writer, I have always put it off. However since going through the coronavirus pandemic and with the news constantly focusing on the negatives, I wanted to offer other sufferers of lyme disease a success story to read for their health battle, to give them some hope. This book follows my journey through my battle with lyme disease, written from my own point of view as a survivor. The statistics recorded in this book are general lyme disease statistics at the time of writing and may be subject to change over time.

For me, the hardest part I found going through my journey was not being able to relate to anybody else and not having something positive to read about people getting better from this awful disease. I truly believe a little bit of hope can make such a difference.

I would never have been able to get through this journey without the love and support the people in my life have shown me, especially my parents, brother, grandma and close friends. They kept me going and fought for me when I didn't have the energy to fight for myself and for this, I will be eternally grateful.

I would just like to thank you for reading my story. It means such a lot to me and I hope it helps to raise a little bit of awareness about lyme disease too.

Jenny

xx

CHAPTER ONE

LYME DISEASE

Lyme disease, also known as borreliosis or the borrelia bacteria which is carried by ticks, is one of the fastest growing infectious diseases in the United States and Western Europe, but there is still so little awareness of it. A lot of people have heard of lyme disease but very few actually know what it is, which is quite frightening considering the severity of it. Unfortunately, less than 50% of people present with the bullseye rash, which can stop people accessing treatment quickly if they don't show symptoms, therefore leaving the disease to manifest into the chronic form.

There are over 300 different strains of the borrelia bacteria, which can affect any and every organ depending on the location of the bite on the body and which co-infections are transmitted alongside the borrelia. The bacteria is circular shaped in structure to protect itself from being killed by the immune system, allowing it to hide and lay dormant within the body. It occurs in different forms and hides in different locations so that it can invade the immune system. It can also change shape and move into different tissues to adapt to the changing environment in order to protect itself from being killed by antibiotics. It is known as a multi-systemic disease which means symptoms come and go in cycles, creating good days and bad days for no obvious reason to the sufferer. Pain and symptoms can migrate around the body and with over 300 different symptoms of the disease, each sufferer presents in a different way depending on their genetics and which infections they have, which explains why it is so difficult to treat.

Many patients become disabled if they are not treated early enough and studies show that they can become just as ill as people who are suffering with chronic congestive heart failure, which is such a scary thought! The average person takes 2-3 years to get diagnosed with chronic lyme disease and if it is left untreated, it can kill you. 75% of chronic sufferers are too ill to work and because UK tests are not sensitive enough to pick up the borrelia bacteria strains, most sufferers are left having to spend thousands from seeking treatment abroad. Unfortunately, I was one of those people who never got any initial symptoms and I don't even remember the time that I was bitten, which allowed this disease to manifest in my body into the chronic form.

I suffered with neurological lyme which means the bacteria travelled into my brain and surrounding tissues, affecting my nervous system. I also contracted two other co-infections through the bite - babesia and bartonella, which are two of the most common found alongside the borrelia. Both co-infections can worsen the symptoms of lyme disease and bartonella can worsen neurological symptoms too.

Babesia was actually the biggest infection causing me problems. Any number over 2 is considered to be a positive result for the infection on the scale and I tested 225! Babesia can significantly increase lyme disease symptoms making a person three times sicker, whilst suppressing the body's ability to fight infections too. It is a parasite and the symptoms are almost identical to those of Malaria. It can intensify and cause chronic symptoms in a person and is considered to be one of the most dangerous co-infections to have as it can eventually lead to heart failure if left untreated. There are also over 100 different strains, with most being missed in Western tests, giving false negative results. Unfortunately this happened to me, I tested negative for all lyme and co-infections on the UK NHS test.

Some of the symptoms that I suffered with were non-epileptic seizures, involuntary and migrating movements in every limb including the face, muscle spasms, concentration problems, mood disorders, sunlight sensitivity, dizziness, lightheadedness, vertigo and balance problems, hallucinations, crawling sensations, heart palpitations, tingling and numbness in limbs, speech problems, insomnia and increased sleep, extreme fatigue, limb paralysis sensations, extreme weakness, air hunger, weight loss, forgetfulness, headaches, exaggerated alcohol effects, flushed cheeks, swollen glands, hot sweats, cold chills, nausea, difficulty sweating during exercise, extreme highs and lows of energy, mood swings, multiple and opposite emotions felt at the same time and body aches.

I've often been told I should write my story and not being a keen writer, I have always put it off. However since going through the coronavirus pandemic and with the news constantly focusing on how many people are dying, not how many are surviving, I wanted to offer other sufferers of lyme disease a success story to read, to give them some hope. I know the hardest part I found going through my journey was not being able to relate to anybody else and not having something positive to read about people getting better from this awful disease. With suicide rates being so high in people living with this disease, I truly believe a little bit of hope could make such a difference.

CHAPTER TWO

LIFE BEFORE LYME

I've always been a carefree kind of girl who loves life and is always smiling. If you ever see me sad then you know something is very wrong! I had such a happy childhood growing up and I consider myself to be very lucky and fortunate with that. I have an amazing family, I had grandparents living close by who were our babysitters when my parents were out at work, of whom I have so many fond memories with. I was shy as a child but never struggled to make friends either. I was such a sporty and active kid, always wanting to try something new and always up for a challenge or a bit of a competition. I guess this competitiveness trait that runs in my family is what helped me get through my difficult years later on. Never one to like being defeated, I had a really strong sense of willpower. If someone said I couldn't do something, I had to try and prove them wrong. Growing up in an extended family with only boys, it was either join them or get left out and where was the fun in being left out? Coming from a medical family too, we were brought up to be tough. If you were sick and needed a day off school, you had to be really sick. I think this is where a lot of my inner strength has come from.

Of course I'd had my ups and downs in the past, I think everybody has at some point or other but I was 22, I'd not long graduated from university with a degree in interior design, which I am so passionate about and I was in my first proper job, finally earning my first real wage. I was fit and healthy (or so I thought), I was going on holidays, partying with friends and living like any other person in their early twenties, generally just loving life!

However, although my health battle felt like it happened suddenly, looking back and reflecting, I guess there was a bit of a build up to that day in November 2013, which I will come to after. Although I perceived myself as being full of health, I guess it actually began to decline in the summer of 2009, the year I left school. I spent the summer mostly outdoors and camping. It was a beautifully hot summer and along with a couple of friends, we were at the end stages of completing our Queen Scout award, equivalent to the Duke Of Edinburgh Gold award, a real privilege to have earnt! We spent four nights and five days hiking 50 miles across the South Downs, carrying everything we needed for the trip on our backs, including our tents, cooking equipment, food and clothes. Halfway up one of the vast hills I suddenly felt like I couldn't breathe. My chest grew tight and I had never experienced anything like this before, but my friends were so supportive and we rested and waited until I was ready to carry on. I was quite scared at the time but I tried to put it behind me and carry on the best I could. The rest of the trip ran smoothly and a couple of weeks later we were going on our last camp with the Scouts before we headed off to university in the September. We caught the ferry over to Jersey with our bikes for a 10 day camping trip. We had such a fun trip and again it was gorgeous weather! We played volleyball on our campsite, went fishing to catch food to cook on our campfire for dinner, we did assault courses and surfing, hiking trips and rode kite buggies. We used our bikes to travel from place to place around the island. I had no problems with any of the activities but once again, several times whilst riding our bikes, I began to experience that same difficulty of catching my breath and a tightness in my chest. The adults on the trip were quite surprised, knowing how sporty I was and so by the end of the trip I had to travel in the minibus around the island instead, no longer being able to cycle.

The September came and off I went to begin my new chapter at university in Southampton. I fell in love with my course and the uni lifestyle, making new friends along the way and joining the trampolining team. That first year had it's struggles as well though. I found out that my gran had got cancer, which was difficult to process being away from home and I also began to experience several bouts of illness myself. I caught several colds, one where my nose was blocked for 10 weeks so I could only breathe through my mouth during that whole time and it took two lots of strong antibiotics to clear it up. Just after my birthday during the second term, I experienced a headache like I have never felt before! My head was searing with pain and I was in bed for three days straight. I couldn't watch the tv, I tried to get up and shower but my head just throbbed too much and there was no way I could turn a light on. I lay there in the pitch darkness, just sleeping as much as I could to try and get some relief from the pain. My boyfriend at the time started to worry about my weight over the next couple of weeks. He had noticed that I had lost over half a stone from the beginning of university and only being a fairly petite person, it was more noticeable. I went to the doctors but he didn't seem concerned so I just carried on with my studies and enjoying the student lifestyle. By the time Easter came around, I caught a chest infection. Back home for the holidays, I went to my GP and got some antibiotics to help clear it up. However, by the time I came back for summer in the middle of May, the chest infection was still lingering so I went back to the doctors for a second round of medication. I enjoyed my summer back at home, going out and about with friends every day and working back at my local job in a bakery where I had worked as a Saturday girl whilst at school.

I went back down to Southampton in the September to begin my second year. I really wanted to start getting fitter again so I decided to try and give running a go, seeing as my new student house was located right next to the vast common that lay at the edge of the city. I had run as a child and I had always had good cardio fitness in the past but now I really struggled to run. My lungs felt like they just couldn't get enough oxygen into them and I'd end up gasping for breath. My chest felt tight and I'd often feel heart palpitations but I was never wheezy. Growing up with a brother who had asthma, I knew it wasn't the same way he felt during exercise but I went along to my local GP to get myself checked out in case. I had to do breath tests over a certain period of time and got diagnosed as borderline asthmatic. I got the inhalers which helped a little but not in the way that I had hoped. Little did I know at the time, that what I was actually experiencing is something called 'air hunger', a symptom of babesia which makes your body feel like it can't get enough oxygen into the lungs.

I carried on the term, with the uni work stepping up a gear but still thoroughly enjoying the student life. However November came and my gran got really ill again, this time nearly on death's door and being rushed to intensive care in a London hospital for a rare blood disorder alongside her second cancer diagnosis. This was a lot to deal with emotionally, especially being 100 miles away from home and my family. The snow hit so badly that year that I wasn't even able to jump on the train to London to go and visit her. The week before I was going home for Christmas, focusing heavily on getting my assignments due in before the break, I experienced burnout. I can honestly say to this day it is the worst feeling. It is so emotionally and physically draining. I like to believe I am normally a very strong person mentally and can deal with everything that is thrown my way, but I was exhausted. I think I cried for three days straight, over anything and everything and nothing in particular. My poor body had being living a student lifestyle of partying, studying hard for a degree, trying to process emotionally my gran's cancer battle, recovering from glandular fever and fighting the early stages of lyme disease, which I had no idea that I had at the time!

Fortunately, the rest of my second and third years at university went pretty smoothly. I studied, I partied, I enjoyed my remaining time in Southampton, travelling to Ireland and Wales for trampolining competitions and to New York with my course friends for a design trip to experience the architecture, fashion and interiors of the beautiful city!

I graduated with my BA(Hons) degree in Interior Design (Decoration) and a month later in July 2012, I started my new job as a visual merchandiser for House of Fraser. I loved it! It was a physically demanding job - heavy lifting, up and down ladders, night shifts, lots of overtime - nowhere near as glamorous as it sounds, but so so creative! I also made some lifelong friends there along the way too. I started off looking after a small section in the store and worked my way up to looking after the whole of the Home Interiors department, designing the layouts of the store's floorplan and creating eye catching displays and windows to entice the customers in to buy the product.

Over that year and a half, although I had recently split up with my longterm boyfriend of four years, I was loving my life! I threw myself into doing a mile swim in the River Thames for charity, I had signed up to a local gym and I was burning the candle both ends, up at 5.30am every day for work but staying out until 5.30am on weekends socialising with friends.

CHAPTER THREE

23RD NOVEMBER 2013

One day, on 23rd November 2013 (I will never forget that date), everything changed overnight. I had been having a few dizzy spells over the last two months but I put that down to long shifts at work and low blood sugars - I'm one of those people that if I need food, I need to eat otherwise I can't function very well. As a child, if I ever got grumpy, my parents knew straight away I was hungry!

I was at the end of enjoying a week off from work after finishing the busy period of launching Christmas. Anybody who's worked in retail knows Christmas is a crazy time! I'd had a fun week off, shopping with my mum, a trip to London with friends and pizza night with the girls. It was a Saturday evening just before dinner and normally I'd have been getting ready to go out somewhere but a bout of dizziness suddenly overcame me. My mum came into the room to find me grabbing on tightly to the kitchen work surface, trying desperately for my legs not to give way beneath me. Being a nurse, my mum checked my blood sugars just in case but everything was normal. So I rested on the sofa and got an early night.

The next day it kept happening, over and over except now it was getting worse. Within 24 hours I had gone from feeling fine to having hot sweats, cold shivers, uncontrollable spasms in my arms and legs, dizziness and collapsing, with all of this happening over many hours throughout that day. Weirdly, I don't really remember being scared. I knew with my mum being a nurse, I would be ok. I had full trust in her that she would know what to do. That evening, we headed over to my grandma's house for dinner. I couldn't get up the stairs to her front door, my legs felt so weak. We phoned 111 and then the next morning I went straight to the doctors to see my GP. I got told they could refer me to get a MRI of my brain done and an EEG, but the appointment would be in four months time. Well, my parents' first thought, not that I knew this at the time, was if this was a brain tumour, I could be dead by then! It's a horrible thought but a true one. To be honest, at this point and throughout the seven years that have followed, I have never really been that scared. Not because I am brave or strong or tough, but because I was just feeling way too ill to even think about what could be wrong with me. I was very much just living in the moment. I didn't have the energy to think about the future. It was a struggle just to get through everyday tasks. I have never been one to take sick leave lightly, it makes me feel guilty for not being able to do the job or task that I was employed to do. I think I had three days off in the previous 11 years throughout secondary school, university and my first part of employment, but I ended up having to go off sick for almost 10 weeks. I tried to go into work for half days sometimes at the beginning, determined that I could carry on living like everybody else but I was so cold I would often wear six jumpers at work and the spasms in my arms and legs meant that I worked a lot slower because I could only use one hand and often couldn't walk properly. My spasms meant that my hand and arm would often get stuck in a particular position for up to eight hours at a time and my leg and foot would turn inwards, making it difficult to walk as I couldn't put my foot flat on the floor. In the end, I just went off sick completely. For those 10 weeks I barely left the house. I was weak, I was tired and some days it was amazing if I could walk to the end of the room without having to sit down and take a rest. I usually needed a nap after taking a shower because I got so tired from the effort of it and a lot of the time I didn't even have the energy to watch tv. I used to just lie there, my whole body feeling like lead and I would have a weird sensation that I felt like I was paralysed. I could lie like that for hours, not sleeping but just having no energy, not even to just move my head.

From being told that it would be a four month wait for the MRI and EEG scans, my mum managed to get me an appointment within the next few days, where she worked at the little local private hospital, to see a Neurologist. The perks of having a nurse for a mum! I know I am incredibly lucky as not many people are that fortunate. They had to pay of course but in their eyes, it was worth it. The doctor's first thought was that it was a neurological presenting symptom, not a neurological cause - something else was going on. Outside of his expertise, he immediately got me an appointment to see an endocrinologist the same night. I was there for about two hours going through every detail I could think of about my life and medical history. The endocrinologist was amazing and I owe a lot to him. I explained that every time I was eating carbohydrates, I was collapsing on the floor, even one tiny spoonful of rice! He suggested I try the Atkins diet for a couple of weeks and see how my symptoms were with that. It was a big diet adjustment but I was willing to do anything just to make these symptoms stop. To my amazement, I felt so much better. Yes I lost half a stone in 10 days but it was so worth it to feel even a small bit of relief from the violent spasms and constant collapsing that were happening on a daily basis. Even my yearly Christmas meal with the girls in early December, all I could eat was turkey and brussel sprouts. It was the blandest dinner I've ever tasted but spending a night with friends was the most joy I ever could've wished for. My friends were honestly incredible. The support I had from them was amazing, I had cards and flowers, puzzle books and other gifts delivered to my doorstep to help cheer me up and they would often pop over to see me if I was up to having a visitor.

However, after a couple of weeks the symptoms came back. I ate dinner one evening, the week before Christmas and the dizziness came back. I fell off the dining room chair onto the floor. I wasn't with it, I was spaced out, I was conscious but I couldn't speak. I kept trying to say words in my head but I just couldn't get them out, there was no sound. My arms and legs started spasming and the limbs were violently flying out in uncontrollable movements. My beautiful dog Twiggy was so protective and came and stood next to me and rested her cheek on mine for comfort. She could obviously sense that something was very wrong. It really is true when they say dogs are mans best friend! She was a great comfort through everything. These spasms and involuntary movements got worse and worse and eventually an ambulance had to be called. The paramedics had never seen anything like it before. I was awake the whole time but both my arms and legs were violently spasming, which I couldn't control. It went on for six hours and by the end I was almost unconscious from pure exhaustion. I felt like I had run a marathon and been hit by a bus 100 times over. I was hooked up to a drip and the doctors came to see me but they didn't know what was wrong with me so they sent me back home.

Back to the GP I went and they ran some blood tests and it turned out I was very deficient in vitamin D and iron, so an intensive course of tablets offered some help with the coldness and severe lack of energy. My days consisted of laying on the sofa and hospital/ doctors appointments for those next 10 weeks. Fortunately, my family were in a position where they could pay for me to see a doctor privately, so I had MRI scans and EEG scans to rule out anything serious.

I took a trip to the Tropical Disease Hospital in London on Christmas Eve. It was a huge struggle getting up there. I was so weak and tired, I had elderly people with walking sticks overtaking me! The reason I went for some tests there was because back in the summer, three months prior to my symptoms, I had swum a mile in the River Thames for charity. Wondering whether I had picked up a parasite after hearing about David Walliams a while back, I needed to rule it out. However all of the tests came back clear, nothing obvious causing any symptoms there. The train ride home was a struggle. Being packed full of people on Christmas Eve, I couldn't get a seat and was slumped over the back of a chair, holding on with every bit of strength I had to stop myself from collapsing. I just needed to get home, I kept telling myself.

On Boxing Day evening, after spending a day crippled in pain and my body twisting and doubled over in positions I have no idea how I ever got into, I ended up back in A&E until the early hours. Once again, the doctors couldn't give me an answer as to what was causing my symptoms so they sent me back home. I went to my GP the following morning and she called the hospital to try and admit me to a ward. I went back to A&E, waiting seven hours to be seen, just to be told straight away without even really being assessed, instead just a quick glance over, that it must be all psychological and to go back home. I was in bits, why did nobody believe me?

New Year came next and desperate to celebrate with my friends, we all went out to a local bar to bring in the new year together. I really wasn't feeling well at all but my best friend helped me do my hair and make up beforehand and when we got to the bar, my friends were all incredible. With my right hand getting stuck in a spasm, there was no way I could hold a drink and a clutch bag. So they took it in turns to help me carry things and when asked by a stranger on the dance floor why my leg was at a funny angle, they all pretended it was a new dance move, so that I didn't feel uncomfortable and singled out. Fortunately, I did pick up for a while after that and after many trips to the hospital and 10 weeks later at the end of January, I went back to work on a phased return. Finally, I felt like I could be semi- normal again!

Around this time, after doing a bit of research on google - I know it's definitely not the ideal thing to do but I did it anyway - I decided to give acupuncture a go. I read that it had many benefits for the body and with nothing to lose, I booked a session. It actually did help to a certain extent. On the really bad days, it helped to lessen the severity of the spasms. I carried this on for two years, starting with three sessions a week and reducing it down to once every two weeks, depending on how bad my symptoms were. But in the end, I stopped going to sessions because my health journey had taken me down another path by that point and I was trialling different treatment options instead.

CHAPTER FOUR

LIVING WITH THE UNKNOWN

At the end of February 2014, my gran had a fall and broke her hip. After battling cancer several times, it was not looking good. She was taken into hospital and then moved to a rehabilitation home and never came back out. The next four months, my own health took a back seat. She was far more important! My poor mum had both of us to look after. Fortunately my health had picked up a bit by then and I was only getting sick for 4-5 days each month, returning to a fairly normal and liveable state inbetween. My gran was amazing, we had a very close relationship and she was like another parent to me. She looked after us when we were kids, she lived a mile down the road and we saw her several times a week. She was the type of woman that would do anything to help anybody. You name it, she would do it! Surprising really, seeing as she had had such a tough childhood herself and no real relationship with her parents, growing up in a children's home during the war. She would give lifts to us grandchildren, did shopping for her stepmother who had once disowned her, lent money to a young boy so he could fulfil his dream of becoming a professional golfer and cooked lunch for me and all of my friends in our school lunch breaks. She was a remarkable lady and I feel very privileged to have had her in my life. By the time June came around, I was visiting her every day after work, in the hospital. It was my time to look after and comfort her in her last days, just like she had always done for me growing up. I made sure I was there right until the very end. After she died, I took it hard. Grief encapsulated me and my health took a decline again. To make matters worse, I found out the day after she died, the man I had been dating at the time had been unfaithful. I felt like my world was falling apart and I had no control over it. I became a shell of the person I usually was. I couldn't eat, I didn't feel like leaving the house and I didn't want to socialise. I had lost my happiness and my spark. My family, my career, my dating life and my health had all taken a big hit at the same time! I had counselling for several months and in the end, I decided to give up my job and hand my notice in. I needed to focus on myself again for a while and it wasn't fair on the rest of my team at work, that I was going off sick for a whole week every month, leaving them constantly short staffed. I felt like I was letting them down and guilty that they were always having to pick up my workload, as I was unable to work overtime or nightshifts or carry the heavy loads as it was a physical job, which came with the job's role. I worked my last day in the middle of September 2014 and the following week I was admitted into Kings Hospital for four days to undertake an epilepsy test. I was hooked up to a machine through 40 wires, all attached to my head and monitored day and night to see how my brain reacted when I had my muscle spasms. Normally I couldn't control when my symptoms would flare up but I needed them to for this test. As food had always been a trigger for me, I ate lots of processed carbs to try and trigger my seizures to help get the most amount of data as possible and sure enough, the large quantities of gluten, dairy and sugar brought them on fast. However, the results came back clear, ruling out epilepsy, which was a relief, but it also meant it was back to the drawing board. From then, I decided to go gluten free as advised by the endocrinologist, as I had been struggling with bloating since the age of 11 anyway.

Once I came out of hospital, not wanting to lose me completely, my manager phoned me and offered me an alternative job on the shop floor as a shop assistant, working part time. I took him up on the offer and did that for the next five months until March 2015. This way, at least I could still earn some money and still be a bit independent. Now only working part time, I decided to enrol on a craft course one morning a week, to give me a new hobby and something fun to focus on. It was beneficial for future jobs as well as it gave me an understanding about how things were sewn for the home. I thoroughly enjoyed the course and it gave me some projects and new skills to work on at home, distracting me from the way that my health was affecting my daily life compared to other people my age, which was really tough to deal with at the age of 23.

After the epilepsy tests had come back normal and I was diagnosed with non epileptic seizures, I then got referred to see a specialist neurologist in the Neurology Hospital in London. I went through all of my symptoms with him hoping that finally I might get some answers! I told him all about the spasms, the collapsing, the involuntary movements and how food seemed to be a big trigger. He wasn't interested in the food at all, to the point where he said to me, "food has absolutely nothing to do with this! You have had some trauma and your brain has learnt these patterns of movements and made them into a normal behaviour for you". A diagnosis called functional motor disorder. He referred me to a cognitive behavioural therapist so that I could have some help in unlearning these patterns of movement. I came away from this appointment so disheartened! My gut, (no pun intended!) was telling me that my endocrinologist was right, there was definitely a link to food and whatever it was, was causing these neurological symptoms as a side effect. However, this was as close to a diagnosis that I had ever had, so I also felt a sense of relief that I could finally put a name to what I was going through, rather than keep having to tell people that still a year later, I simply did not know.

That Christmas, I started a whole new chapter in my life. My mum had inherited my gran's flat after she died back in June, so I moved into the flat with my best friend, just before our 24th birthdays. I was so excited to finally be living independently again, as I had moved back in with my parents after finishing university and I was so excited to be living with my best friend as we had known each other since we were at nursery school. We had been through everything together and our relationship is so strong, we are basically like sisters. I couldn't wait for all the new memories we were going to make together! One of the biggest things I've struggled with through my whole seven years of illness is constantly feeling like I'm in a bit of a limbo stage and falling behind where other people my age are in life, not having reached where I thought I would be by this point in my life. I imagined after leaving school I would fall into a career and work my way up the ladder but in reality, my career has taken a big hit. Don't get me wrong, I have put everything I possibly could into my career but the obstacles I have had thrown my way has altered my direction in ways I have had no control over, so I have just had to do the best I could. Maybe I'm being too harsh on myself but if you don't have goals, then what drives you forward in life?

I began a month's worth of CBT sessions with a doctor in London but I hated them. I've never been one to talk a lot about my feelings, I suppose mainly because I don't want to burden anyone. I am such a happy person by nature, I don't want to talk about negative things and I certainly don't want to make anyone else less happy by bringing the mood down. However, later on in my journey, I discovered this is not a healthy approach to always have. Sometimes you have to face your problems in order to free yourself so you can move forward. During CBT I learnt several grounding techniques and every time I was having a non epileptic seizure, I would try and focus on different senses such as smell and touch to focus my awareness and try to stop the movements becoming so bad. It didn't really work and I never really tried using the techniques for long after my sessions came to an end, if I'm honest.

Another memorable night for me was my 24th birthday. I was known by all of my friends to be quite a party girl, not the biggest drinker but always on the dance floor and the last one to leave to go home. I've always just loved the feeling of letting your hair down and having fun with friends, not a care in the world in that moment of time! During the early hours of the morning, a large group of us waiting for taxis to take us home from London, something in me just switched. At the time, I had no idea what was affecting my mood. Always the calm and laid back person, I suddenly felt myself getting angry. I argued with my friends and this was so out of character for me, people were shocked. We got in the taxi and I half fell asleep, although it was mainly the drowsiness of a seizure coming on. By the time we reached our flat, I couldn't get out of the taxi. I just couldn't make my legs work properly enough to walk. My best friend's boyfriend had to carry me into the flat and I managed to stagger to the sofa. Moments later I had fallen off the sofa onto the floor in a full seizure, fully aware the whole time what was going on but so tired from the night of dancing, the alcohol I had drunk and the energy being used during the seizure. I knew they were both scared, as I think it was the first time either of them had seen a bad episode like this and so they called my parents at 3am, who took me back to their house to look after me for the next few days. Staying at my parents' house became a regular thing over the next few years. Once a month on my bad days, I would go over to their house to be looked after until I was well enough to go home and do things for myself again.

By the time it got to March 2015, I was still struggling with taking a lot of time off sick, even just working part time hours so I decided to hand in my notice again, for good this time and concentrate on myself for a while. As much as I wanted to work, I now knew that health is the single most important thing in the world. Without it, you can't live, it's as simple as that. So I joined a local health club where I could use the gym for gentle exercise and the sauna and jacuzzi to relax in after bad symptom days, to try and keep my body in as healthy state as I could, despite whatever was going on inside! Whatever this was, I knew I needed to be as fit and as strong as I could possibly be, if I was to ever get better and recover. I took on some voluntary work on my good days, helping to paint theatre stage sets for a local company, so that there weren't too many gaps in my CV and also took on two zero hour contract, admin type jobs over that summer so that the days when I was feeling good, I could still earn some money and get out and about and live my life as well as I could, keeping my independence.

My endocrinologist had done everything he possibly could for me within his field of expertise by this point and I was finding it really tough that I kept getting told my condition was psychological by all of the other doctors. I had been referred for yet more CBT to deal with chronic stress. I kept trying to tell people that I was only feeling down as a result of my symptoms, my symptoms were not a result of me being depressed. I persevered with the CBT sessions but I found they had no real relevance; I couldn't relate to anybody in my group who were mainly suffering with anxiety at work and nobody could relate to my situation either. So the endocrinologist referred me to a private nutritionist in London, with a clinic on Harley Street, who dealt with unexplained illnesses. Finally I had some more hope and meeting her turned out to be the best thing that has ever happened to me. This first appointment in June 2015 also turned out to be the pivotable turning point for the beginning of my road to recovery! I owe her my life as I know it now and I genuinely don't think I ever would've recovered without her. Armed with my full medical history right from when I was in the womb, information on all of the milestones in my life and details about the relationships with the people around me, I headed up to London for my first appointment. I was greeted by a woman with the warmest personality and the most knowledgable mind in her field of work. Working with patients across the world, if anyone could help me, it surely had to be her! She told me about her own previous health battles and we had such an in-depth conversation about mine, lasting almost two hours. It was worth every penny! She believed me about food and diagnosed me with SIBO - Small Intestine Bacterial Overgrowth. Basically this is where bacteria from the large intestine moves up into the small intestine where it isn't supposed to be, causing all sorts of digestive issues. I was to begin a low fodmap diet straight away, eliminating all the foods that were more acidic and harder to digest and eating mainly alkaline foods. The idea was to try and starve and kill off the overgrowth of the bad bacteria, relieving the symptoms. This was really tough, it meant cutting out dairy, gluten, sugar and a lot of simple every day foods. Restaurants for me, instead of being a place with a menu full of choice on tasty things to eat, have become a menu full of food items where I have to scan so thoroughly to find something on there that I actually can eat. However I still love eating out, it's such a lovely social thing to do with friends and loved ones and now that allergies are higher and veganism is more popular, it is slowly getting a lot easier. I lost a lot of weight in a short time after I first started the low fodmap diet and went down to my lowest weight since being an adult. Now a size 4-6, I was bordering being underweight and a lot of my bones were showing. I was put on a lot of supplements to make sure I was still getting all of the nutrients that my body needed but I felt so much better! I had some withdrawal symptoms to begin with, headaches and food cravings, but by eating healthy and nutritious meals, I was no longer getting the mid afternoon slumps of energy and found being on a higher protein, low carb diet worked so much better for me energy wise, once I had adjusted.

I headed off to Ibiza with a big group of friends for a week in the August and had the time of my life! Sunbathing, water sports, pool parties, clubbing, what more could you want?! I was 24 and back to loving life! I mean I wouldn't quite say I was back to normal, I went away with a bag full of medication and had to watch everyone else eat all the tasty things in restaurants that I couldn't, but surely that was a small sacrifice to make? Anything to me was worth feeling back to my happy and positive self again, like I had been when growing up. I slowly began to reintroduce foods one at time over the coming months, learning which foods were triggers for my body. After the Ibiza holiday though, I decided to give up alcohol for the foreseeable future. I had a taste of what living symptom free was like again and I wasn't going to let anything ruin or take that away from me.

In the October, I got my first job as a junior interior designer! I was finally doing what I loved and was using everything I had learnt in my degree. It was a small local company, I had my own office and I began to work on some amazing projects. I had meetings with suppliers, attended trade shows abroad in Frankfurt and Paris, discovering the latest design collections from around the world. It was my dream job!

2016 came and generally it was pretty smooth sailing health wise. I say that, but I was still going off sick for three or four days every month, it would take me about a week to recover fully from the fatigue, but then I was managing to live a pretty normal life in the weeks in-between. I was 25 by this point and really desperate to feel like I was still able to achieve things, despite my limitations. I decided to write myself a bucket list of 30 things I wanted to achieve by my 30th birthday, which to this day I am still working towards, with the 30th birthday looming closer! It gave me something positive to focus on, which has really helped me mentally.

In the February of 2016, one of my friends moved to Australia for a year to go travelling. It was a bit of a gamble for me health-wise but myself and another close friend decided to plan a three week trip to go and visit her over the following Christmas and New Year. It was a once in a lifetime opportunity that I did not want to miss or regret, so I took the plunge and booked it. The worst that could happen was that I would get ill for a few days and have to stay in bed. I had been dealing with these symptoms for three years by this point, so I knew exactly how to cope and although I would be the other side of the world from my family, I had full trust in the girls that I was holidaying with, that I would be safe.

That summer, myself and four other friends I knew from school, travelled out to Prague for a girls holiday to watch our other friend get married. It was such a lovely day, the sun was shining, the venue was gorgeous, the bride looked beautiful and the whole trip was full of laughter from the day we got there to the day we left. Travelling for me in general hasn't been easy. It takes a lot of mental energy as well as physical energy and it would be a lie to say that I wasn't a little nervous beforehand, on all of my trips. It takes a lot more preparation because I have to make sure I have medical notes with me as I have to carry a separate hand luggage bag just for my medication. I also have to think about food and taking snacks with me as finding food abroad can sometimes be tough, depending on the country. I would often have a flare up of symptoms in the days following my holiday, just from the sheer exhaustion and the mental strain of desperately trying to stay well throughout and enjoy my time away.

When I got back from Prague, another thing on my bucket list was to start a new hobby. I started aerial hoop classes and it has honestly been one of the best things I have ever done! I get to relive my acrobatic days of being a gymnast when I was child. The instructors and girls there are all amazing and it is very sociable, having yearly dinner and dance balls, aerial performance shows and charity events. I have met some incredible girls there that have become such close friends too and always offer amazing support.

Around that same time I also met my new boyfriend who quickly became my rock. He never knew me before my illness but that didn't phase him at all. I was incredibly lucky to have him in my life, especially through what was to become my most difficult year at the end of 2017.

I contracted a kidney infection in the September 2016 which escalated pretty quickly and within a couple of hours I had to go to A&E for antibiotics. I ended up having two courses to clear it up and at the same time, I also tested positive to having a parasite in my body, so I had a course of treatment for that as well. I began having a few sessions of IV vitamin and magnesium infusions during those next couple of months too and I think all of this treatment combined, killed off enough of the lyme bacteria to temporarily give my body a boost. It gave me a couple of months break from having any symptoms, which was a miracle, as it meant that I was able to get through my once in a lifetime trip to Australia, completely symptom free! So on 18th December, we headed to Heathrow Airport to begin our adventure, both of us so excited and my parents left at home worried sick that I would be ok, should anything happen!

Armed with three weeks worth of medication, enough snacks to try and last me as long as possible and sacrificing a hairdryer for a handheld blender so that I could at least make a nutritious breakfast smoothie each morning before trying to find food for the rest of the day, we jetted off. First stop was Singapore and we spent the whole two days non stop sightseeing in the glorious heat. Unfortunately, Singapore was not good at all for gluten or dairy free eating, so I barely ate whilst I was there. Safe to say by the time we arrived in Australia on 22nd December, I was absolutely starving!!! We spent a couple of days in Perth visiting family friends and exploring the west part of the country before heading up to Cairns to meet our friend who was travelling. It was the best reunion! We stayed there for six days over Christmas, where we cooked a traditional english Christmas dinner and watched a festive film, we sunbathed, we partied, we explored the rainforest, met real aboriginal people, had a go at spear throwing, boomerang painting and snorkelled in the Great Barrier Reef. We then flew down to Sydney to spend the next week and to bring in the new year. We ended 2016 with a helicopter ride over Sydney and watching the spectacular fireworks display. We watched an opera at the Royal Opera House, we fed kangaroos, visited the Blue Mountains, climbed the Sydney Bridge, surfed on Manly beach along with many other amazing experiences. It was an emotional goodbye, before flying to Hong Kong to spend a couple of days there on the way home. Looking back, I can't quite believe I managed to get through that whole trip feeling as well as I did and I can't be more thankful for that!

Unfortunately, a couple of weeks before our Australia holiday, my beautiful greyhound Twiggy had to be put down. I was completely heartbroken. We had had her for nine years and she had been through everything with me. School exams, boyfriend breakups, family bereavements, starting new jobs, university and all of my bad health so far. She left a massive hole in our hearts and our lives. When I got home from my Australian trip a few months later, we decided to re-home another rescue greyhound. That's when Molly became the newest addition to our family. She was beautiful and such a mischievous dog but also so affectionate that you couldn't stay mad at her for long! She was also very intelligent as dogs go and was always making us laugh on a daily basis, something which was a huge support for me particularly on my difficult days. The first half of 2017 I had a lot of fun. I was going to the gym regularly, I was enjoying my aerial hoop classes, I had so many things planned with my boyfriend, family and friends; weddings, hen parties, my grandma's 90th birthday, day trips to London and the coast and exciting projects at work. I was enjoying my life. For every bad day that I had stuck in bed each month, I was certainly making up for it on my good days! However life did always feel like a bit of a risk. I loved to plan social things and book events but at the back of my mind, there was always a chance that I may have to miss it if I fell ill. It felt like my life always had an air of uncertainty about it. I tried my best not to think about it, to only worry about being ill if it happened, which for me was the best way to cope. I tried not to dwell on the feeling of constantly being different to everybody else my age. I was still going to enjoy my twenties, no matter what obstacles were thrown at me. After all, you're only young once and you never get that time back!

CHAPTER FIVE

RECEIVING A DIAGNOSIS

In the May I caught a stomach bug. Now everybody knows just how awful you feel with one of those but when you have an underlying chronic disease like lyme as well, your body and immune system simply just cannot fight hard enough. Any other illness I caught, I always got it worse because it would cause my lyme symptoms to flare up as well. I remember for several days, heaving and throwing up, my stomach was so swollen I had severe sharp pains and I looked like I was nine months pregnant. All of my limbs were in pain and I felt so restless. I just couldn't get comfortable no matter what position I was in - lying down, sitting, standing. I felt faint, I felt like I had electrical currents running through my body and the only relief I could get was when I was asleep. Fortunately this only lasted about five days in total but of course it brought on the muscle spasms and non epileptic seizures for a couple of days too.

By this point, I still actually didn't know that it was lyme disease that I was dealing with. I had been working with my nutritionist for almost two years by this point and although my SIBO had improved dramatically, I had hit a plateau and I should have been showing more progress. This is when she said to me there must be something else underlying and that she was going to send for every test she could think of until we found out what was wrong. I can never be thankful enough for her persistence to never give up on helping me. Not actually thinking it would be lyme disease because I didn't present with the typical symptoms, it was a shock to discover that that was what I had. I had neurological lyme, which is a slightly rarer/ more unusual case of the disease. Well at this point I had no idea what lyme disease even was, I had never heard of it! I had such a mix of feelings; a great sense of relief in that finally after three and a half years I had a definite diagnosis but that I was also about to enter a new chapter into the complete unknown. With my nutritionist not being a specialist herself in lyme, we then had to do a lot of research ourselves into finding the best treatment plan and doctor. That was a lot of pressure when we knew nothing about it. My first action was to ask my GP to do a lyme disease test for me on the NHS to see what kind of treatment was on offer down that route, but the results came back negative. In England, the chronic form of lyme disease does not exist as a medical illness yet, they simply do not have the funding to do the research into it. It is fine if you catch the disease within the first eight weeks of being bitten by a tick because a simple blood test will show up the infection and a short course of antibiotics can treat it. But the trouble is, tick bites are often so small, sometimes as small as a poppy seed, that you can't see it attached to your body and less than 50% of people actually get any kind of symptoms after being bitten. If you're one of the unlucky ones like me, it can go several years undetected in your body, lying dormant before any symptoms begin to show. After those initial eight weeks from being bitten, the bacteria of the disease very cleverly moves out of the bloodstream and hides inside the cells in your body so that NHS tests no longer show that you have the disease. It is also a great imitator, mimicking so many other diseases like MS and fibromyalgia, that people often get misdiagnosed with other illnesses. The bacteria can also change form so that it becomes resistant to medications, meaning it is difficult to treat.

After receiving a negative result through the NHS, I still needed to find a treatment plan and a doctor. I had a couple of options, there was a new private lyme disease clinic opening in Southern England in the next couple of months but did I want to be one of their first patients and potentially be one of their trial cases? This wasn't particularly appealing to me as I wanted somebody I could put my full trust in, who had a high success rate. Bearing in mind there is no test available yet that can guarantee a 100% recovery for lyme disease, we are still too early in medical research for that, I wanted somebody who could treat me so that I could live my life symptom free again. The next option was a private clinic north of London who had treated some cases but there were mixed reviews about it. Another option was to travel to America to one of their lyme disease clinics but America seemed such a long way to travel, especially if I would have to go there multiple times. It would also be costly as my family were going to have to pay for all of my treatment themselves, which has turned out to be thousands! Luckily I knew somebody that had a family friend who worked for a lyme disease charity here in the UK and who had suffered with lyme disease herself. She was able to give me lots of information on where people had found the best treatment as well as give advice from her own experiences. She was living a symptom free life now and she had been treated in the BCA Lyme Disease Clinic in Augsburg, Germany, the very place where I had sent my test to, to get my diagnosis. My mum had also bumped into the endocrinologist who had treated me in those years before and although he didn't really know much about lyme disease, he had heard of the BCA clinic in Germany too. So that was sorted, my decision was made that I would travel to Germany to begin my treatment. They offered a three week intensive programme with two lots of tests beforehand and then patients were able to travel back home, providing the doctors were happy with the progress made, to carry on the treatment back in their own countries. I booked my first trip for the initial assessments in the September and booked the intensive treatment programme for the October. I was excited but nervous as I was finally going to be able to treat this once and for all, but I was also nervous because I had no idea what to expect. Naively, I thought I would be 'cured' by the end of the three weeks and would be able to live a normal life again once I came home. I couldn't have been more wrong if I'd tried!

The first six months of 2017, Molly our new greyhound had been a big joy and comfort to have around, helping me especially through my illness. She was such an affectionate dog, always wanting cuddles and strokes and I honestly think she thought she was a lap dog, despite weighing 24kg! She was so mischievous as well, often stealing shopping bags, shoes, clothes, cushions, anything she could pick up and take to her bed. If you told her off for sitting in an armchair, you'd soon find her sitting in another one, as if to say, "well you didn't say I couldn't sit in this one!" She was very partial to any food that was cooking as well. She once tried to steal my lunchbox off the table very slyly when she thought I wasn't looking. Although she was mischievous, she was gradually learning what was deemed acceptable behaviour and what wasn't and with a bit more training, she would've flourished! Heartbreakingly though, we discovered a lump on her stomach, four months after we rehomed her, which turned out to be a cancerous tumour. We bandaged up her stomach every day to stop the bleeding from the tumour, for as long as she was still living a happy life and enjoying her walks. On 3rd July, just six months after rehoming her, she took a turn for the worse and we had to have her put down. We were completely devastated. Even just a short six months, she left a huge gaping hole in our hearts. We'd lost our two beautiful dogs within just eight months of each other which had a huge impact on my mental strength, coping with my illness. There was no longer a happy dog there wagging her tail and trying to cheer me up with cuddles and laughter on my really difficult days, when I was struggling to get through just simple everyday tasks.

During that summer before I headed off to Germany, I actually had a holiday booked in Rhodes with some of my close girl friends from school. I had been looking forward to it for so long! I had never been to Greece before, it was going to be a new country I could tick off my bucket list and I couldn't wait for some girl time and lots of sun, sea and sand. However in the days leading up to the holiday I was getting worried. I could feel my typical lyme symptoms coming on, which often felt like I had electric currents running through my limbs and I just knew it would be such a struggle to travel abroad if I was having lots of spasms and involuntary movements. I just had to get there! But I also didn't want to be ill once I got there either. I came home from work the day before we were due to travel and my mum came over to my flat to see me. I burst into tears, what was I supposed to do if I got ill on holiday? I knew my friends would have been amazing no matter what happened, I fully trusted them 100%. They had been through this illness with me by my side for the last four years and two of them had been my friends for over 20 years. I just didn't want to ruin their holiday as I couldn't live with the guilt of that! My mum told me the worst that could happen, would be that I would just have to sit by the pool for a few days or rest in the apartment and actually was that such a bad thing? Probably not really! Armed with a big bag of epsom salts in my suitcase, to help calm my muscles if I were to get any spasms, along with extra magnesium tablets, I jetted off with the girls. I honestly don't know how I got through that holiday without getting ill. I guess it was the extra high doses of magnesium and sheer willpower and determination to enjoy my week in the sun, have a break from work and enjoy some time with the girls that got me through! I always had to be careful though, more sensible than I sometimes would've liked to have been! I could never fully let my hair down because I knew at the back of my mind I needed to keep that balance of not overdoing things or exhausting myself too much that would've brought the symptoms on. I couldn't drink on nights out, which was sometimes very tough, particularly when others were but fortunately I'm quite a night owl so I'm good at staying up late and I love a party. Even when I'm sober I love to dance, which definitely helped me to still enjoy nights out. I just had to make sure that I didn't compromise on my sleep too much and make sure that I didn't go long periods without eating either. I could have fun as long as I was careful too, not something you always want to hear in your mid twenties, but it was the only way I could live my life in the most enjoyable way that the disease would allow. Luckily I did mange to enjoy my holiday and to get the break that I really needed because I was not prepared for what I was about to come home to! Sure enough, with the sheer relief of getting home having survived the week without any symptoms, I was able to relax fully and then the lyme symptoms began the next day. I was in bed for several days with the spasms, seizures, collapsing and constant fatigue and when I returned to work, I got hit with the bombshell of redundancy. I was not at all prepared for it. I also endured a nasty comment from my boss's partner about my low weight, something which was very sensitive to me at the time as I had struggled to keep a healthy weight throughout my battle, despite my sheer hard work of eating healthily to manage my digestive issues and keeping strong and fit through exercise. The comment hurt. I had generally had a good relationship with my boss throughout my employment there, despite often having to fight the company's corner through issues with clients and suppliers. Things quickly turned sour over the legalities of redundancy and I ended up having to take him to court. The last thing that I needed was a court case when I was about to start treatment in Germany and I think he knew this too. Still to this day, I am owed a lot of money from him but in a way he did me a favour by letting me go, as I would not have wanted to have been caught up in a business like that from the things I learnt about how it was being run. It also then gave me the time I needed to really put my health first and concentrate on beating this nasty disease once and for all!

CHAPTER SIX

BEGINNING INTENSIVE TREATMENT

October 12th 2017 came and I boarded the plane to Germany with my mum. I felt such a mixture of emotions. Excitement to finally be starting treatment, apprehension as I had no idea what to expect, sadness at leaving my boyfriend behind at home for the next three and a half weeks and also guilt that I couldn't be at home to support my brother, who was moving back in with my parents because he was having marriage problems. I knew he had my dad there for support but it was still hard.

In the days leading up to our flight to Germany, I had been having some spasms in my arms and legs. I knew more than anything that I just needed to get out there! I also knew my mum was worried but adrenaline took over and we made it to Augsburg with a pretty smooth journey. Arriving fairly late in the evening, our first task after settling into the apartment was to find a nearby restaurant that catered for my gluten and dairy free requirements. With neither of us having learnt any German before, google translate and google maps soon became our saviour. How did we ever cope without them? Our apartment, home for the next three and a half weeks was only half a mile away from the clinic I would be having the treatment in and it was located on the 15th floor of a tower block, offering the most beautiful panoramic views of the city in the changing autumnal season and showcasing the most spectacular sunsets I have ever seen!

The next day we took a walk down to the clinic so I could have some blood tests and scans done, to determine what state my body was in prior to starting the treatment. It only took a couple of hours and the test lab was in the same building, so by lunchtime we were free to go. Although being October, the weather was so beautiful, about 22 degrees which certainly put a positive light on the reason for being there. We spent the rest of the day exploring the town as you do being a typical tourist and we stocked up well on food! We then had the whole weekend to sightsee before my treatment began on the Monday morning. This was my favourite part of the trip and fortunately I was feeling well enough to see everything that we had planned. I knew I would feel worse once the treatment started but I wasn't prepared for just how much worse, which makes me all the more grateful for that one final weekend of enjoyment! We caught the train to Munich for the next two days where we explored authentic German markets, climbed the Bell Tower, took a city sightseeing bus tour, explored the local parks; bustling with people playing games, riding their bikes, busking with their musical instruments and we visited the Dachau Concentration Camp which was such a eye opening and harrowing experience but so worth the visit. We then finished the days with a meal at the Hard Rock Cafe - I try and visit them in every city I go to and of course finding a gluten and dairy free pizza too, forever my favourite food!

Monday 16th October 2017 - the day my treatment started, almost four years after my first seizure and worst symptoms had begun. It was a journey that had been a long time coming! I was nervous going to the clinic that morning, it felt like the first day at a new school or job. I didn't know anybody and I didn't really know what to expect or what challenges I was going to face. The only comfort was I knew this was my chance for a road to recovery. My mum was of course with me but it was very tough for her too. She wouldn't be able to come into the treatment rooms with me so it was unfair to make her sit in the waiting rooms from 8am until 4.30pm every day, that would have been so boring! It was also tough for her as we were in a foreign country, neither of us knew the language or anybody else and she was alone every day for those three weeks while I was in the clinic. Fortunately the weather was fairly pleasant at the beginning so she could go for walks each day around the town and local parks and she basically became my personal nurse and carer for the duration of the stay, cooking the meals, cleaning the apartment, washing our clothes and doing the food shops. She had worked a lot of overtime in the months leading up to the trip so that she was able to take four weeks off work to come with me and I will forever be grateful for that, along with everything else my parents have done and sacrificed for me. It's a debt I will never be able to repay!

The intensive three week programme consisted of treatment from 8am to 4.30pm, Monday to Friday and during these three weeks we were hooked up to IV antibiotics for three hours every day. This was so that the body could get a higher dosage of the medication, with less strain and more protection on the stomach and digestive system - especially as some of us had digestive issues! It also allows higher levels of the antibiotics to be absorbed by the body. This part of the day was a chance to get to know some of the other patients in the clinic. There were up to 10 people being treated each week but although we were all battling lyme disease, our symptoms were very different. We all sat opposite each other, with people ranging from 18 years old to their late 70's and all from different countries around the world, therefore all speaking different languages! This proved a slight problem but luckily for me, English is a widely known language. It was the first time in my whole four year battle that somebody could relate to what I was going through. It was such a massive comfort, I can't even begin to describe and still to this day almost three years later, I keep in loose contact with two other girls from other countries, to see how their treatment and road to recovery is going and more importantly, to offer each other support when it is needed and celebrate those little victories that are accomplished! The IV was hard, some days it would make me feel sick, sometimes it would cause a drop in blood pressure and it was also tough on the veins with needles being stuck into them every day. We often had to rotate veins between the ankles, elbow creases and back of hands so that they didn't get too bruised. Not to mention the tough challenge of actually having to sit there for three hours not moving the limb which had the needle sticking in it which is not easy when you're a naturally active person!

We were all given our own little boxes to carry around the clinic with us, containing things we would need for the treatment. I don't know whether this was deliberate or just coincidence as German words are translated differently, but we were all given lime green blankets for when we got cold, something which is very common in lyme sufferers. Lime green for lyme patients, it gave us something to laugh at anyway!

Alongside the IV antibiotics we had to undergo several holistic treatments each day, the idea that these would help push the antibiotics into every single part of the body and also help to eliminate any toxins being released. We had to get our bodies into an alkaline state, trying to avoid any kind of acidic levels because this would stop the disease from spreading. A really important aspect of starting treatment was focusing on our diets. Again, we had to focus on eating alkaline foods and avoiding acidic ones, so we were given a long list of foods and their quantities that we were allowed to eat and we had to cut out dairy, gluten and sugar, as the disease thrives off these foods. Fortunately, I had already been doing this for the last two years which unknown to me at the time, explains why I had started to improve so much when I started working with my nutritionist and why I was managing to live a fairly normal life in-between the flare ups. It had also given me a massive advantage in that my body had already done a lot of preparation work prior to starting the treatment, meaning that I could tolerate the treatment a lot better. The other treatments each day included:

- Light therapy - sitting in front of a UV lamp for 30 minutes. Light therapy helps improve sleep, helps strengthen the immune system and helps to reduce depression/ low moods which are all side effects of lyme disease and are all so important in improving health.

- Magnetic Fields therapy - sitting in essentially what is like a massage chair, sending vibrations around the body at a specific frequency in order to push the antibiotics into every part of the body. It helps improve circulation in the body, activates the body's metabolism, improves oxygen levels in the blood and helps to strengthen the immune system.
- High Tone therapy, a similar experience to magnetic fields, except the vibrations cannot be felt. It involves pads being attached to the wrists and soles of the feet for one hour, helping to reduce energy blocks in the body and relieving any pain.
- Oxygen therapy - sitting on a bike pedalling for 20 minutes with an oxygen mask on, which helps to improve the efficiency of the antibiotics by increasing circulation. This also in turn helps to reduce any side effects of the medication.
- Exercise - 45 minutes in the gym, either cardio or weights with a personal trainer tailoring the exercises specifically to each patient. Exercise helps to decrease inflammation and increase detoxification of the body, helping to also move the antibiotics around, reaching more cells. It also boosts energy levels and mood as well as increasing the body's strength and range of motion.
- Heat therapy - sitting in the infrared sauna for 20 minutes to sweat out as many toxins as possible. The heat helps stimulate circulation, relieves pain and again strengthens the immune system.

As the days went by in the clinic, I was becoming weaker and weaker. When you have the chronic form of lyme disease, the bacteria hide in the individual cells in your body. The treatment works by bringing the bacteria out of the cells and back into the bloodstream in order for it to be killed off, essentially poisoning your body in the process. The reason it is the worst known bacteria to mankind and the bacterial disease equivalent to cancer is because it can very easily become resistant and transform. This is why no singular drug can kill it off. Multiple and very strong medication is needed for there to be a chance of killing it. In my case, I was on four very strong antibiotics all at the same time; Atovaquon/ Quensyl used to treat malaria, Eremfat used to treat tuberculosis and two other very strong ones called Minocycline and Cotrim. That is why the side effects can become so severe.

By the end of the first week the fatigue was beginning to set in. I definitely didn't have the same level of energy that I had had the week before. However, being encouraged by the clinic to keep exercising every day to keep the oxygen flowing around the body, we headed into the town of Augsburg where we were staying, to do a bit of sightseeing. We went to the local zoo where I had to sit down half way round, but it was a great place to visit and gave us something enjoyable to do after a week of being in a hospital. We also visited an old self-contained village where some religious people still live today, costing them only one euro a year to rent their houses.

The second week of treatment, I began to feel worse and worse and by the next weekend, I was starting to feel really rough. We only managed a small walk around the park next to our apartment each day and the rest of it was spent on the sofa watching Netflix. I expect it was highly boring for my mum but she said she didn't mind. Into the third week of treatment, the walking to the clinic each day was becoming harder because I was really struggling for energy and there were days when my right leg began to spasm and it was getting weaker and weaker, meaning I was constantly having to sit down on a wall for a break, my mum linking my arm so I could put some of my weight onto her. But I had to keep going. I'm so glad at this point that I didn't know it would be eight months before this right leg gained back it's strength again! Exercising in the gym was becoming harder too. I was limping on the treadmill because my leg was just so weak, it was giving way under my own bodyweight and weights were becoming harder too because the strength I needed to lift them was fatiguing my body so much, it was causing my limbs to spasm. However I just had to grit my teeth and get on with it. I couldn't let this disease win and defeat me. How else was I ever going to get my life back otherwise? I just put my full trust into the doctors and trainers, they knew what they were talking about, they were the professionals.

The staff at the clinic were all amazing and so friendly. The clinic itself has been treating patients for over 20 years and only treats lyme disease and it's co-infections. Many of the staff and doctors themselves have had lyme disease in the past and are now recovered and helping all of us on our journeys too. I was also having to take other medication during seven different times of the day, to help supplement vitamin deficiencies that were caused by foods cut out of the diet and from the disease itself. To put into context how difficult this disease is to treat, I have been on about 70 tablets a day for the past five years. I have a cupboard at home that is purely designated for medication. I guess to most people that probably sounds awful but to me it has just become a way of life, I actually feel strange if I don't take medication (in the few times I have to come off to do tests) and actually, it has given me my life back so I don't associate it as a hard or difficult thing to do. It's become a bit of a laugh with my friends when I always request the allergy menus and then bring out the pot of pills on the table in restaurants.

November 3rd 2017, we were finally flying home. It had felt like we had been away a lifetime! I couldn't wait to see my family, boyfriend and friends again. To say the trip home was exhausting would be an understatement. I generally believe it was one of the toughest experiences of my life! With extreme fatigue, a right leg that I couldn't put weight on, an arm that was in constant spasm, you don't realise how far the distances through an airport are until faced with those limitations! My mum had to carry both of our suitcases the whole way, heavy from a three week trip abroad and try to support me with my walking at the same time on the long journey home of a train, a plane, and another train before my dad picked us up. It was nearing midnight and with a slight slope at East Croydon train station up to the ticket barriers, I honestly felt like I was trying to climb Mount Everest! What would normally take me about a minute to walk, took me almost 10; I was holding onto the rail with every ounce of what little strength I had left in me, not to collapse on the floor. It sounds pretty dramatic but I am not exaggerating. It's a feeling that I can't describe, it's a different type of exhaustion and pain that only comes with a chronic illness. Wow was I glad to be home!

CHAPTER SEVEN

THE UPHILL CLIMB

Little did I know, things were about to get a whole lot worse! Back at home I was to replace my IV antibiotics with oral tablets instead and to carry on exercising as best I could and going in the sauna as much as possible, which I luckily had access to at my local gym. Then I would retest and speak to my doctor in eight weeks time, the middle of December. Fortunately I have never had to go back to the clinic as they have everything set up so well for people to carry on treatment from other countries. They post me over a blood test kit which I take down to my local GP surgery, they carry out the test, give it back to me and then I post it back to the labs in Germany where they process the results. I allow two weeks for the results to come through, before discussing them with my doctor via telephone or Skype. I can then order my new medication through the clinic's website and they get posted over to me from Germany to the UK, often arriving within a couple of days. Although it has been expensive because I had no option but to go private for all of my treatment, it has been worth every penny for the service and treatment I have been given and for getting my life back!

It was pretty lucky actually that I had been made redundant just before I flew out to Germany to begin my treatment because it took the pressure off feeling guilty about getting better quickly enough to get back to work. This way my health became my priority and I could let it take as long as it was going to take! It was now the beginning of November and I couldn't wait to see my family and friends and of course my boyfriend again. It had been about a month since I had seen them all and also another priority since being home, was to find and rehome a new greyhound, something that our family were so desperate and excited to do! That's when Leo joined our family and he is the most loveable and adorable dog and so affectionate. He wanted so much attention from us all, lots of cuddles and playing together with toys and he also had the mischievous side that Molly had had too, often stealing my towels when I was running a bath and wasn't looking, or stealing tea towels and clothes, or even one or two cushions! It always gave us something to laugh about every day.

The winter months came so I didn't mind spending time indoors but I was finding the more I was going through my treatment, the worse I was getting. I hated having my independence taken away as it meant I was having to rely on other people to help me, which is something I was not very comfortable in doing. The downside to taking such strong antibiotics was that I was plagued with yeast infections over the next eight months, the only real time in my life that I have ever suffered from them. I was no longer having all of the supplementary therapies but I was making sure I was still getting exercise every day and trying to use the sauna at my gym as much as possible, along with epsom salt baths at home. My walking was getting worse and worse because the treatment was making my right leg weaker and weaker. By the end of November my boyfriend suggested to me about using crutches. I hadn't actually thought about that but it was one of the best ideas! I just used one crutch to help support my right leg but it certainly helped with my independence and it helped me move around a little bit quicker as well. It meant it was easier to meet up with friends, get around the gym and get on public transport. It also made other people aware, that although to them it probably looked like I was injured, it meant people would give up seats for me (most of the time) on transport or hold doors open for me, just little things that made all the difference. At the beginning of December, my boyfriend flew out to Australia and Hong Kong for a three week holiday to see family. It was tough mentally because not only had we spent the whole of October apart, we were now having to spend December and Christmas apart too, at a time when I probably really needed him the most. But that's the way life goes sometimes and he was still an incredible support to me, even from the other side of the world. He had such a great sense of humour, always making me cry with laughter, so he definitely helped to keep my spirits up during my most challenging times.

I had to have regular blood tests and ECGs to check my heart during those first weeks back at home, to check that everything was going to plan. I had my eight week review via telephone with my doctor in Germany at the beginning of December to discuss the results and I had had big hopes of coming off the antibiotics then. No such luck. Although I was definitely improving, the lyme and co infections were in no way gone. I still had work to do yet. I was disappointed but in actual fact, this is totally normal for patients with chronic lyme, it is not a quick road to recovery at all. I just didn't know that at the time!

January 2018 was definitely the hardest and most challenging month of my entire life to date. What I had to endure is actually quite difficult to put into words. To explain the medical side, when a patient is undergoing lyme disease treatment, in order to get rid of the disease out of the body, the antibiotics work in a way that extract the bacteria and parasites out of the cells and tissues that they are hiding in and bring them back into the blood stream. The process in which this happens, means the body is effectively being poisoned during this time. So obviously with me having lived with the disease for so many years, it was a tough process and there was a lot of the disease to kill off. This also creates a lot of inflammation and toxins in the body, which can temporarily worsen the symptoms of the disease, known as the Jarisch-Herxheimer reaction (shortened to herx reaction) named after Adolf Jarisch and Karl Herxheimer. Luckily for me, my boyfriend had returned from his three week trip abroad just in time to spend New Years Eve together, full of laughter, fun, food and games with some of our friends. A couple of days later, my leg spasms began to get even worse and I was struggling to walk, even with the crutches. I phoned my parents and they came to pick me up from my flat and I went and stayed at their house so they could offer help if I needed it. I ended up staying nearly four weeks! What came next was the worst time of my life. The Herxheimer reactions I experienced were horrific, I never could have been prepared for them but I just knew that I had to keep going and get through it if I was to ever get better. I had severe muscle spasms in almost every limb of my body, sometimes muscles getting stuck in certain positions for up to eight hours at a time, or sometimes moving so uncontrollably I just became exhausted. My body would twist and turn into such awkward and bizarre positions and sometimes I would fall off the sofa onto the floor and wouldn't be able to do anything to stop myself. The violent spasms spread to my face which would sometimes make it very difficult to talk and eat. I tried to keep my spirits up by joking about the funny facial expressions I would make because if I didn't laugh, I would cry and crying wouldn't help keep my strength up to fight. I was also collapsing several times a day, even with the crutches. I never lost consciousness when I collapsed but I always struggled to talk. I just couldn't get any words out, no matter how hard I tried. I always went drowsy too but could hear everything that was being said around me. Typically I would come around within about 15 minutes or so. It became such a normal thing in my family because this happened so regularly, that as mad as it sounds, sometimes family members would just leave me to it until I called them to say I was ready to try and get up and needed their help. Often I preferred it this way, the less fuss the better and they couldn't really do anything to help me anyway. It was just a waiting game. There were many times over that month that the spasms in my hands were so severe that I had to get my parents or my boyfriend to feed me. Sometimes I was so drowsy or my mouth was in spasm too that it became very difficult to eat or chew. My body was so weak that I would sometimes just lie on the sofa for hours, not even watching tv or doing anything, just lying motionless staring into space because my body was so exhausted and felt like it was in a state of paralysis, that I simply did not have the energy to do anything. I often needed help getting dressed, going to the toilet, getting in and out of the bath and had to be carried to bed every night. For being such an independent person all my life, it was really tough mentally to deal with needing this level of help to perform basic tasks in my mid twenties. I felt worlds away from everybody else my age living their lives. I would often suffer with brain fog as well, a common symptom of lyme disease and would regularly forget what I was saying midway through a sentence or I would forget very basic words which could be so frustrating. With my stubborn nature and my willpower to get better, I would do everything I possibly could for myself. If I wanted a cup of tea, I would attempt to make it myself before asking for help, even if it meant making it one handed, painfully slow and nearly spilling it several times trying to drink it. Anything I could do to stay independent I would do. I think I was quite frustrating to my family in that respect because I often refused their offers of help! Strangely, I also remember I had such strong cravings for ready salted crisps the entire time too. I would often get through family sized bags of crisps on a daily basis, not very healthy I know, but at least they were still gluten and dairy free and being borderline underweight at the time, the extra calories were probably a good thing! Being housebound for almost the whole month of January had a huge effect on my mental health because I became so frustrated that I could barely do anything for myself and I also became claustrophobic being stuck inside the same four walls day in and day out.

By this point, it had only been two months since we had rehomed our new greyhound Leo. Having a dog there for comfort in the past, to cuddle and make me laugh particularly during flare ups, I was hoping for the same with Leo. However with being so ill, our relationship took a big hit. Understandably I think he became wary of how I was behaving. Obviously seizures, collapsing and violent muscle spasms are not normal behaviours and I think he often mistook my muscle spasms for me being angry and tense which made him very unsure, especially in a new environment so he would often growl or bark at me if I tried to stroke or cuddle him. This greatly upset me at the time because I needed the comfort more than ever but looking back I can completely understand it from his point of view. We are very much friends now and our bond is so strong. I can happily say he never growls at me anymore and welcomes as much attention and fuss from me as he can possibly get!

As another method of support during this time, I started going for regular reflexology sessions with one of my neighbours. I find the sessions so good for me, both physically and mentally. It's a time I can completely switch off and relax but the therapy also helps to support the systems in my body and keep them balanced from the side effects of the treatment. My neighbour is one of the most caring people I know and never fails to make me laugh. I love our catch ups during our sessions and she's become a great friend.

By February 2018 I was starting to feel a little better. I was going to the gym on crutches with my boyfriend and my brother and they both helped me build back up some strength. I was so weak that I could only manage 1kg weights to begin with but the feeling was so good and it was great to see some of my friends there again too. I was still learning the fine line between trying to exercise but not overdoing it and one night I obviously pushed myself a little too hard and I couldn't stand back up from the mat. My legs would just not move and when I tried, I collapsed back to the floor. My boyfriend had to carry me down the stairs, out to the car and take me home but it was a good lesson learnt. You don't know much you can do unless you try! As much as January had been the worst month of my life, when I retested for the lyme and co-infections in the February, the lyme was in a negative state - I couldn't believe it! All that pain and suffering had been worth it and that only strengthened my determination to get better even more. I still had a long way to go though.

I decided as I wasn't working that I would do some courses in my field of work to help me when the time came for applying for new jobs so I signed up for a course in Sevenoaks, a train and a short bus ride away. I managed to get there ok on my first day but coming home I could feel my symptoms beginning to start again. It took me a while to walk to the bus stop on my crutches and I had to sit down on the pavement while I waited as I was running out of energy. The bus driver was so kind to me and gave me a free ride to the station. I was desperately trying to hold back tears and I just wanted to get home. My family and friends were all working as it was the middle of the afternoon and there were no cabs available in the area for quite some time. I got to the station and a man who worked there also helped me down the stairs and onto the train. I was trying with every bit of energy I had to stay upright and not to collapse by this point. Eventually I made it back and my dad picked me up from the train station. Although the lyme disease had gone into a negative state, it didn't mean every single trace of it had gone yet. It was going to take a while for my body to recover with everything it had been through! I managed to get through the rest of the course without a glitch and I soon signed up to another three day course in London at the end of the March. The course was so worth it and I thoroughly enjoyed it. However by the end of the third day, the physical stresses on my body of learning something new and travelling up to London took their toll and unfortunately, not everyone on public transport was kind enough to give up their seats, despite seeing me standing with crutches. My dad was picking me up from the tram station and by the time I got there, a few minutes early, I was struggling not to collapse. I managed to lower myself to the ground and sit on the pavement while I waited but not a single person stopped to ask if I was ok. By the time my dad arrived, I couldn't stand back up, I just didn't have the energy so he had to lift me into the car and back out again when we arrived home. That weekend was actually the last of my severe regular spasms and collapsing. I gradually began to improve day by day and began to get stronger and stronger, so much so that by the time the London Marathon came in April, I managed to travel up to London to support a friend who was running in it. I managed to walk six miles around the city on the crutches which was such an accomplishment! Of course I was extremely tired by the end of the day but I was so happy that I had been able to go and support him.

But then another blow came. Out of nowhere my boyfriend and I were forced to break up. We had been talking about marriage and children but unfortunately we came from different religious backgrounds and once the Church had found out he was planning to propose to me, they forced us to make an impossible decision and only gave us a 24 hour time period to do so. We were so in love and it had been the best chapter of both of our lives together, but we were in a lose-lose situation. We either had to give up a part of who we were individually or we had to give up each other. As devastating as it was, we both wanted each other to stay true to who we were because they were the versions of us that we fell in love with, so we parted ways. I lost my partner and my best friend over night and out of the previous relationship breakups I have experienced, this just didn't even compare. I was completely and utterly heartbroken. I actually felt like I was grieving a death rather than the loss of a relationship because we didn't part through a loss of love, so I couldn't have any bad feelings towards him. But I also knew at the back of my mind that I had to keep being strong at the same time in order to keep going with my treatment and to get better. This had to be my number one focus and priority now. It took me a very long time to move forward from it and work through that grief but I did learn to accept it and was able to move forward and I have now found a place of happiness and excitement for the future again and to see where my life is going to take me. One of my close friends, who I met on a work trip to Germany a couple of years earlier, also went through a breakup at the same time so we jetted off to Ibiza in early May for a girls holiday and some much needed fun!

CHAPTER EIGHT

LIFE AFTER LYME

At the beginning of that June I was finally able to stop taking the strong antibiotics because the hardest part of killing the disease was done. I also had become strong enough to walk unaided and decided to ditch the crutches which was such a huge achievement and milestone! I was starting to become a bit bored and restless being at home so I decided it was finally time to start looking for a new job. It had been eight months since I had worked and I was so ready for a new challenge. I got offered a job with a small local company at the beginning of July as their junior interior designer and I absolutely loved it! My team were fantastic and I still consider them all to be friends today. They took a big risk hiring me considering my past health and sickness records but I was honest with them from day one, which they hugely respected and said they were willing to take the risk. I was hired on an initial one year contract just in case it didn't work out health-wise. I only worked part time, starting at reduced hours three days a week, increasing up to full days and then up to four days a week. It was perfect for me and I gained so much valuable knowledge and experience.

Over those next six months, I continued focusing on working hard to heal my body. I made sure I kept my stress levels as low as possible, I prioritised my sleep and I made sure I was getting 7-8 hours every night. I kept strictly to the recommended dietary plans and kept my heart rate below 130 during exercise. I found that when building up my strength, I had to work harder to get the strength back in my right arm and right leg where I had suffered with the majority of my muscle spasms over the years. I also suffered with weak ankles from a lack of cardio, which I needed to build back up too, to help with my walking. I continued to get better every week and I was finally managing to get my life back on track, living relatively symptom free. I was building up my fitness levels and I finally got back to my aerial hoop classes after eight months too, which was the most amazing feeling ever. I absolutely love it, it's my happy place! I had a small relapse just before the Christmas where I experienced a few muscle spasms in my right arm and leg again, where I think I had stressed my body a little too much. Being Christmas I had relaxed my diets slightly, had been fighting a cold and had been working a few more hours finishing off a project in time for the Christmas break but a few days rest and I was feeling so much better again. Although the relapse was disappointing, I had just survived nine months without any seizures, spasms or collapsing and I had recovered pretty quickly, so I knew I could do it again. I was learning my body's limits and no road to recovery is ever a straight line, there are always bumps along the way!

Throughout 2018 and 2019, my lyme disease tests kept alternating between borderline and negative, meaning that although my symptoms were so much better, there were still a tiny few traces of the bacteria left in my body, ready to flare up symptoms when my body went through times of stress. I improved greatly from the rest period over Christmas and I came back fighting even stronger than before in the new year. My fitness was improving in the gym, I was out having fun with friends and I was gradually increasing my hours at work which was all such a positive step forward. I started dating a great new guy and we had a lot of fun together. Sadly, after four months we split up due to other things going on in life. We parted on friendly terms and I respect him for the choice that was made but I was still upset. The same week my lyme disease test came back positive again which was hard to deal with mentally after having worked so hard the last year to get better. It felt like a step backwards. Two weeks after that was my review at work as my initial one year contract was coming to an end. We had agreed soon into me starting there that my manager would renew it no question, as we worked so well together as a team. But unfortunately the company had hit some tough times financially and I was called in one lunchtime at the beginning of July, to be told that she had to let me go and couldn't renew my contract. Two of us were made redundant that day. With the contract finished, I wasn't entitled to any notice or extra pay, so I finished that day. It was a huge shock because I had had no time to prepare. I hadn't been able to save any money and suddenly I was left without a job and with no money coming in. I didn't blame my manager, it was just a difficult position to be in. To make things harder, my best friend, whom I had been living with for the previous four and a half years, was moving out two days later as she had just bought a house with her boyfriend. So I was going to have double the amount of bills to pay, although my parents helped me out and I was about to start living on my own. It was an incredibly emotional time her moving out because it was the end of a chapter for both of us. We have been best friends since we were two years old and have been through everything together. The day she moved out we both cried and it was a strange feeling walking back into the flat on my own with all of her things gone and an empty bedroom. But at the same time I was so incredibly happy for her and her boyfriend and their exciting new chapter together. She deserved it and I was such a proud friend.

It was a lot to process in such a short space of time; my health, my home, my relationship and my job. I felt like my world was falling apart around me. A few days later I suffered another relapse of my seizures and muscle spasms, which I am almost certain was due to stress. I began to feel more and more tearful which was so unlike me because I'm always such a happy person. I got an interview for a job a week after that, which I was really excited for and pinned a lot of hope on but sadly the competition was too strong and another candidate was a better match for the role. I was gutted. From then, my mood was getting lower and lower and I was beginning to struggle to find happiness in things. Even my aerial hoop classes which I absolutely love, I wasn't finding enjoyment in anymore. By the end of July I hit an all time low. Many days I would wake up and just not want to be here. I felt numb. I wasn't exactly suicidal, I didn't actually want to die, but I felt like I was drowning and that I needed a break from life. I stopped going out with friends for a while and I became so quiet when I was around people. It was a particularly tough time because five of my close friends were moving in with boyfriends over that summer so they were all having incredibly exciting times and of course I was so incredibly happy for them too, they all deserved it, but selfishly it was also a reminder of everything that I was losing as well, which I hate to admit. My friends were all so amazingly supportive through it all, especially a few close friends in particular and I can't describe how much it meant to me to have them there. I managed to get a zero hour temporary job back at the opticians where I had worked four years previously, which definitely helped me to get out of the house and distracted me from everything that was going on around me. Just a few short weeks later, at the beginning of August, my brother, just turning 31, began experiencing awful headaches and his eyesight suddenly turned to double vision. He had to go for some hospital tests and they found a shadow on his brain. As a family, we are such a strong unit but we all fell apart that day. It is the only occasion apart from a couple of funerals that I have seen both my parents cry. The pain we all felt that day was awful. We had no idea what this shadow was but the first thought was a brain tumour. We had to wait three whole weeks to get the results of this shadow, living in this horrible limbo period of not knowing, millions of thoughts of what ifs rushing through our brains. My heart ached for my parents, having both their children going through such horrible health experiences. I can't begin to imagine how they felt, let alone how they stayed so strong.

I decided at this point that I needed to seek some professional help and I was diagnosed with Post Traumatic Stress Disorder (PTSD). I suffered with depression and panic attacks over that summer and began having counselling. Throughout my whole health journey, I had always been so open about everything that I was going through and was able to talk about it very freely but suddenly I couldn't talk about it anymore without getting upset. Apparently this is often pretty common with chronic illness sufferers - they focus so hard on getting through and dealing with the physical side of the illness, that it's only when they are finally better, that the emotional side catches up and needs to be dealt with. Counselling was the best decision I ever made. I went every week for three months and I can't believe how much of a difference it made. There were many things that I had bottled up and never really confronted or dealt with and the weight that was lifted when I did face them and learn to grieve for them was remarkable! I soon got my spark, my drive and determination and love and happiness for life back again and in the October, I started a new job working with such a lovely team of people at a great company. It is also my first job working full time since my health took it's turn and I had to resign from a previous job back in 2014. Since then, my brother's shadow thankfully turned out not to be a brain tumour but it is thought to be MS instead. However with slowly improving symptoms, this cannot be officially diagnosed unless another bout occurs. My lyme disease tests have continuously stayed negative and I have had no more relapses, now being symptom free for a whole year. I feel better than I ever have before and I finally feel like there is light at the end of the tunnel and I'm beginning to close this chapter and put it behind me. I am looking forward to a bright and healthy future ahead of me and I am so excited for it. Something at one point, I never thought I would have. Although I have now received two negative lyme disease tests in a row and have been completely symptom free for a year, and another year before the mini relapse, I am not quite there yet but I am on the final hurdle and I'm certainly moving forward with my life and putting it all behind me.

Lyme disease affects the immune system, preventing it from having a long lasting functional antibody response. It goes deep into the tissues in the body where it's harder for antibiotics to reach. The CD57 white blood cells which help to fight infections are lowered, particularly in people with neurological symptoms, making sufferers even sicker. Still to this day, although I no longer suffer with lyme or co-infections, I am still working on building my CD57 cells back up to a normal level. Unfortunately I have been left with a little permanent nerve damage from the lyme disease in my right arm and right leg but I am slowly learning how to recognise it and how to live with it, so that I don't really notice it as much anymore. It's a small price to pay for everything that I've been through.

Since treating the lyme and co-infections, my SIBO has greatly improved as well. I still suffer with a lot of bloating and pain and travelling really disrupts my digestion as well but I am learning what foods are triggers for me. I still follow the low fodmap diet too but I have slowly introduced a lot more foods back into my diet over the years and I can now eat a greater variety which is good. I have become so in tune with my body that I know what is normal for me and what isn't and it's taught me so much about the importance of health, diet and nutrition, a topic I have become so interested in. Our GI tract houses about 80% of our immune system so if our digestive system is functionally poorly, so will our immune system. SIBO can also cause a lot of inflammation in the body which is why it is important to follow the fodmap diets in order to heal. The testing for SIBO isn't the easiest, it can take a lot of mental energy to complete. The actual test itself only lasts a couple of hours and involves breathing into a test tube every 20 minutes after drinking a sugary solution, to monitor how the digestive system reacts to it but the hardest part is the preparation beforehand. It involves a 24 hour period of only eating plain white rice, baked chicken or turkey and plain eggs along with drinking water. Aside from being boring to eat, it can often cause headaches as well. This is then followed by a 12-16 hour fast before the tests begin. Fortunately I only have to do these tests a few times a year!

Alongside this, I have suffered with mould toxins in my body. Mould is a neurotoxin and can alter the normal activity of the nervous system, contributing to and worsening neurological symptoms in lyme sufferers. It also has immunosuppressive effects and can affect concentration levels too, something which for me, still hasn't fully recovered yet. My nutritionist and lyme doctor believe this could be the cause for my still suppressed CD57 levels, so I am currently going through a detoxing treatment programme to get rid of the mould from my body. On the days I take the medication, I feel very fatigued, sometimes nauseous, very bloated and headachy, but this is all typically to be expected as the mould is being killed off and toxins are being released into the body so reducing inflammation as much as possible is needed.

Despite having beaten the lyme disease and co-infections, I am still currently taking about 70 tablets a day to support my health. I cannot be discharged from the BCA Clinic in Germany until my CD57 cells have increased so I am still on medication from them to help support my immune system. I am also on medication to help with the SIBO to support my body with nutrients and vitamins that I may be missing from a more restricted diet and also if my body is not absorbing them from food properly yet, as well as to help reduce the levels of inflammation that SIBO can create and finally medication to kill off the mould in my body. Alongside the medication, I carefully monitor my diet, exercise and sleep to keep my body in a state of optimum health, in order to be in the strongest position that I can be, to fight off any infections and regain my health. I also have monthly reflexology sessions to help support every system in my body and keep them functioning as best as possible, as well as regular massage sessions to release toxins from the body, keep muscles performing well and reduce any inflammation. I use infrared saunas at my gym a couple of times a week and I take regular epsom salt baths because magnesium is calming and is a muscle relaxer, as well as being necessary in over 300 detoxification reactions in the body.

At the beginning of the year, I experienced my first winter cold in six years that didn't trigger any lyme disease symptoms, which for me has been such a huge milestone. It reinforced to me that I am finally getting better and all my hard work over the previous years has been worth it. I also went on to receive the 'Most improved student in Aerial Hoop' award which meant so much to me. It was another reminder of how hard I have worked and that anything can be possible when you set your mind to it. There were many times over the past years when I wanted to give up and trade my body in for a new one that 'worked properly'. Having lyme disease has put my body through so much, it blows my mind how it can even begin to recover but I'm so glad that I have never given up. Now, I am managing to hold down a full time job, exercise 4-5 times a week and go out and about with friends and family, socialising and travelling. It's strength, determination and willpower that has pushed me through and got me to this point.

Although not considered a high risk during the Covid19 pandemic, I am still considered a higher risk than other people my age due to my immune system not having fully recovered yet. I decided at the beginning of lockdown, that if I was unable to work for the foreseeable future until things are safe again, I didn't want to waste my time off during furlough. My health was going to be my number one priority and I have been more determined than ever to push through this final hurdle to regaining my health, especially with the pandemic being a reminder of just how important health really is in life! I have had the chance to really focus on the mould detox programme and also with the gyms closing, it has been a great opportunity to focus on my cardio stamina, something which took a big hit over the previous years, with having to keep my heart rate below 130 in order to keep my body in an alkaline state. I decided to take up running and with never really having run much before in the past I set myself a challenge to reach a 10km. I am so proud of myself at having achieved my goal and it made it feel even better that I achieved it in the week of exactly two years after learning to walk again unaided, following the eight months of using crutches. I can feel myself getting stronger every day.

It's also given me a chance to reflect and think about what else I want to achieve in life. I know I want to help people in some way and I hope by writing this, I am able to give other lyme disease sufferers some hope for the future in their own health battles. I have no idea what lies ahead of me but I do know that I will always vow to myself to stay strong and happy and I'm looking forward to even brighter days ahead!

CHAPTER NINE

THE EMOTIONAL EFFECTS

I think my journey through my health battle has actually affected me emotionally more than I consciously realise. Everybody has always said the whole way through how strong I have been, which honestly is the biggest compliment I could ever receive. I actually think maybe the reason I have appeared so strong is because I have blocked most of it out of my mind, which isn't necessarily a good thing. I have a very strong habit that if something doesn't make me happy I will block it out and box it away without really confronting it, which is probably why people rarely ever see me feeling down. Sometimes this can be good and it definitely helped me get through all of the bad days because I just kept focusing on and living for the good days. However there did become a point where it all got too much when I suffered with the PTSD in the summer of 2019.

Some things throughout my journey that have impacted me emotionally and mentally, I have got through and some I am still dealing with. Initially, I used to get embarrassed about my involuntary movements and muscle spasms in public, in fear of people looking at me differently but it actually didn't take me long to not care about that because the people that knew me, gave me so much positive support that actually it didn't really matter what strangers thought about me. I was never going to see them again so why should I worry about their opinion? It grew my confidence dramatically and I'm really proud that such a negative experience of having a chronic illness has caused such a positive change in my life. I used to feel guilty for cancelling on friends when I wasn't well and feel guilty for spending days on the sofa just watching tv but I used to say to myself that I wasn't being lazy, I was just on my 'energy saving mode'. My body and my health and the rest that it needed to heal and recover was my number one priority and other people would understand that too and if they didn't, then they weren't worth being friends with anyway! I also used to get embarrassed ordering food in restaurants because in most places, instead of scanning the menu with so much choice for what to order, I tend to have to search the menu trying to find one dish that I can actually eat without it causing me to feel unwell. Often I will have to adapt dishes and it always takes slightly longer to order with the waiter which means that sometimes more focus is on me. It used to really annoy me when waiters thought I was being fussy because I didn't 'like' a lot of food, which is actually completely the opposite, I love food and would give anything to eat the large choices available! But I soon got over this too. Again, why did I care what a waiter thinks? They aren't an important person in my life and why should I let anything stop me enjoying a social occasion with family and friends? Now I always sit in restaurants with my little pot of tablets out on the table, ready to take with my food. I don't care what other people think of me, I am who I am and I can't change what has happened to me.

I have never really questioned "why me?" or felt that it was unfair that this has happened to me either. In actual fact, it's given me a new perspective and I often think to myself that I have been fairly lucky. Far worse things happen in life and there are a lot of things that I would find so much harder to deal with. It's something that has happened, that I cannot change, it was out of my control, so why waste precious mental energy on feeling sorry for myself or focusing on the past? I have a roof over my head, I have access to food, I have been able to work and earn money, I have the most amazing support network of people in my life, I have access to hospitals, I have my sight, hearing, speech and my limbs - yes they have been effected but only as side effects from the disease. All of this alone makes me a lot more privileged than a large amount of the world's population, so everything else in life is just a bonus really. I shouldn't be complaining!

Although I said that I have learnt not to care about what other people think of me, particularly strangers, I still do struggle a little bit with how to approach the subject with new people in my life, people that I have met since my poor health began. I struggle because they didn't know what kind of person I was before my illness, so mainly I don't want them to see me as being weak, but I think the biggest thing, is I don't want to become known as the 'girl with lyme disease' or the 'girl who is ill'. I want to be known as me, for being me, with my illness just being a part of what I have been through. It's that fine balance of needing to make them aware without it becoming a big thing, especially when conversations come up about food and eating out together, why I have so many tablets I have to take each day or why I have had so many jobs in the past or why I can't push myself in exercise to the same exertion point that a normal person can. I have always been so open and honest about my whole journey and I will always answer any questions that people have about it, but at the same time, it's not really a part of my life that I want to focus on, it's a time that now I'm almost out the other side, I want to put behind me so I can move forward.

Another way it has affected me mentally is the constant feeling that I am behind in my life. I think one of the hardest things was seeing my friends all progressing in their careers after finishing university, which is an opportunity that I have not been so fortunate to have had. Don't get me wrong, I have tried my absolute hardest to maintain a job as much as I can but my career is probably the area of my life that has suffered the most. I was simply too unwell to hold down a full time job for about five years so it has meant that I have had to work part time, take time out from work completely to focus on treatment, change jobs frequently - not helped by two redundancies! - and have had to stay in more junior roles while I gain the experience.

Another thing that I never talk about is how my weight changes have effected me mentally. I lost a lot of weight in the first couple of years, dropping from 9 stone 3lb down to 7 stone 10lb, partly because of the restricted diets I was having to follow to stop the symptoms from flaring up but also because the disease itself was stripping me of a lot of the vital vitamins and nutrients I was eating from food, limiting my body's ability to absorb them. I became used to looking at an undernourished and underweight version of myself. Since beating the disease and getting it into a negative state in my body I have naturally put on about half a stone, which is a better weight for my height. I know it is a good thing and everybody now says how well and healthy I look and that I have my sparkle back in me. They are right and I would 100% rather weigh a bit more and be living a healthy disease-free life any day, but I have still had to adjust to seeing my body a bit bigger again. I am in no way unhappy when I look in the mirror because I know how strong my body has had to fight to get me back to being healthy again and I will always love it for that. I train really hard and eat really well and really look after my body to keep in good health, which definitely gives me body confidence but I do have days when my SIBO flares up or on certain days during my menstrual cycle, where I can suffer from extreme bloating, sharp pains and I can look about eight months pregnant, which can be extremely uncomfortable and give false body image views in the mirror. However I just have to remind myself what I have been through, how far I have come and to be kind to myself. My body has achieved incredible things, it's never going to be perfect, but then whose is? It's much more important to have a strong, healthy body, a life that I love and be beautiful on the inside, than to have a body that simply looks good.

I suppose if this was going to happen to me at some point in my life, then it happened at the best time. Although it did disrupt some of my young years, I had already managed to gain my degree and finished all of my studying. I had already got one foot in the door to begin my career, even though that has been affected. I was lucky enough to have moved out and live independently but without the worry of paying a mortgage or feeding/ looking after a family and children and I was young enough that I had the best chance of fighting and beating this disease. The older you are, the harder it is for your body to fight it so by judging all of that, I consider myself to be pretty lucky!

I try not to think about what could have happened if my family couldn't have afforded the treatment - probably in a wheelchair and bed bound with no job or social life, no sport, no independence, purely a matter of existence rather than living a life.

I've always been a great believer in life that everything happens for a reason. I don't know the reason why this has happened to me, I guess it was just a case of very bad luck which I've accepted. Instead, I can try to use this experience in a positive way. Although I would never have wished this to happen to me - or to anybody else for that matter - if somebody asked me would I change my past, the answer would be no. I certainly would never want to relive my journey and yes I would've saved myself from a lot of pain and difficult struggles and experiences that I still sometimes struggle to think about now, but it would've meant that I would never have become the person that I am today. I never would've fallen back in love with fitness the way that I have, I never would've met some of the amazing people I have met along the way, who I am so lucky enough to call my friends and I never would've gained the inner strength, determination and willpower that I have today either. I know that anything thrown my way in life I can deal with and that one day things will get better. Nothing, no matter how good or bad, lasts forever. I have truly realised what is important in life. I have a newfound love and respect and appreciation for every single person in my life. It has brought me out of my shell and turned me from a shy child into an adult who loves to meet new people and learn about their stories and what makes them who they are. I never judge anybody in life because you just simply don't know what battles they have had to face and I truly never ever take anything in life for granted either. Health is the single most important thing in life, without it you simply cannot survive and what gets you through the tough times is the people that you surround yourself with. They are the people that will fight for you when you don't have the energy to fight for yourself. They are what keep you going and I will forever be eternally grateful for all of the love and support the people in my life have shown me, especially my parents, brother, grandma and close friends. Words will never be enough to describe how thankful I truly am to them. I can now say writing this, I am finally back to the fun loving and carefree girl that I always used to be, just a much stronger and wiser version! Lyme disease has shaped me into the person that I am today, it's a part of me that I can never change but I will never let it define me, because if I do, then I have let it win and being the competitive person than I am, I will never ever let that happen!

ABOUT THE AUTHOR

Jenny Hodges has always been the kind of girl who loves life and is always smiling. She lives and works in London, close by to where she grew up with her family. At the age of 22, her life as she knew it was quickly turned upside down with what would turn out to be a seven year long battle fighting lyme disease and other health conditions. This book documents her journey navigating life with a chronic illness, taking her down paths she never expected to take. Determination and willpower has pushed her through the fight for a diagnosis and the gruelling treatment programme that followed, giving her a whole new perspective on life. Always looking for the positives in every situation, being defeated was never an option for her.

Printed in Great Britain
by Amazon